7 Reasons to

Skin Brush Every Day

Improve Circulation, Digestion, and More!

Albi Hamilton

November 2014

What is Dry Skin Brushing, Exactly?

Have you seen those brushes in the "spa" aisle at the store? They have wooden handles and natural bristles, they are usually about 9-12 inches from one end to the other, with the head of the brush (where the bristles are), being about 4-5 inches long and a couple inches wide. You may have wondered what those are for, who uses them? Are they for scrubbing in the shower? Are they to be used while in the shower, while wet? Technically they could be used in the shower, but they are called Dry Skin Brushes. They were believed to have been originally used by Japanese for thousands of years, who induced vigorous scrubbing with loofa sponges before their hot spring baths.

Later, Scandinavians and Russians using dry skin brushes similar to our skin brushes of today, combined massage and skin brushing with little nodules on the opposite side of the head, to be used for a type of slightly more aggressive massage. These types of brushes were pounded onto the guests in spas of places like Baden-Baden, Germany for at least the last few hundred years. The idea behind this type of brush is to break up the toxins within the capillaries next to the skin so they may be carried away via the lymph fluid through the vessels and off to the lymph nodes (our bodies have three times more lymph than blood).

Today this combination of massage and skin brushing continues in a segmented population of spa culture, and has most recently been infused with salt-glow therapy, which is discussed briefly later in this book.

How Does Dry Skin Brushing Work?

Dry skin brushes are usually made of natural fibers, often times from a squash. When choosing a skin brush, make sure to get one that is non-synthetic fiber. Also, a long handle is good for reaching all the areas of your body, and try to find one with bristles that aren't too stiff, but also not too soft.

When people talk about dry skin brushing, they are referring to using this dry, natural bristle brush in a specific pattern in an effort to do two things:

1. Stimulate the lymphatic system
2. Remove the skin of dead skin cells and other material clogging the skin.

The lymphatic system includes lymph fluid, special filters called lymph nodes, and a network of capillaries and vessels that carry the fluid through the body. Skin brushing literally moves the lymph through the capillaries, to the vessels and nodes. The particular pattern used in skin brushing is essential because since the lymphatic system has no pumping mechanism of its own, this pattern is meant to serve the purpose of following the path of excretion from the body.

Lymphatic Cleansing Through Dry Skin Brushing

We have all heard about the lymph nodes, but what else do we really know about the lymphatic system? What does it do? How can we take care of it? These are big questions that are best answered thoroughly and revisited frequently, because we all know it isn't easy to schedule in time to take care of ourselves. But we need to do it, right?

Dry skin brushing is one of the fastest, simplest and easiest way to stimulate the lymphatic system, because most of the capillaries of the lymphatic system are near the surface of the skin. Of key importance is the understanding that the lymphatic system *doesn't have* a pumping mechanism of its own- therefore each stroke of the skin brush has more of an effect on the movement of lymph fluid throughout our bodies that we often realize.

Why Do We Have a Lymphatic System?

The lymphatic system carries toxins from the outside world, such as microorganisms and other living particles,[1] as well as byproducts of joint and muscle use (biochemical waste), such as arthritic and lactic acids, away from the cells of the body.[2] Our bodies have three times as much lymphatic fluid ("lymph") as blood.[3] The lymphatic system is an open system that is a part of the circulatory system, which is the largest system in the body. Over 20 liters a day of blood are filtered through the capillaries, vessels, and nodes of the lymphatic system.[4] Lymphatic capillaries "are small vessels located in the spaces between all cells in the body, except the tissues of the central nervous system and non-vascular tissue."[5] Lymph consists mainly of lymphocytes, which are white blood cells (T-

---

[1] National Cancer Institute.
http://training.seer.cancer.gov/anatomy/lymphatic/
[2] National Institute of Health.
http://www.ncbi.nlm.nih.gov/pmc/articles/PMC2755111/
[3] Hagerup, A. http://ezinearticles.com/?Understand-Your-Lymphatic-System-and-How-to-Keep-It-Healthy&id=5230977
[4] Wikipedia. http://en.wikipedia.org/wiki/Lymphatic_system
[5] Medical News Today.
http://www.medicalnewstoday.com/articles/272054.php

cells, B-cells, etc.). Blood and lymph flow together at one stage, and later the two separate, with the red blood cells (RBC) going one way and the lymphocytes, plasma, debris and pathogens being carried in another direction. The colorless lymph fluid is filtered in the nodes and later excreted in normal fashion (yep, you know what *that* is), but because the lymphatic system has no pumping mechanism of its own, it relies on gravity, muscle movement through exercise, dry skin brushing, massage, and deep breathing -such as in yoga, Pilates, and meditation, for circulation of the fluid throughout the body. A healthy lymphatic system has the added benefit of keeping the body "regular."

A Sluggish Lymphatic System is More Common than We Realize

Blockage can occur within the lymphatic system when infection from debris or pathogens, such as bacteria and viruses, are building up at the site of the nodes. This condition causes buildup in the surrounding tissue, or lymphedema. From sinus pressure, frequent headaches to weight gain and fatigue, a variety of common ailments in our modern society can be attributed to a sluggish lymphatic system.

Essentially, many other systems of the body, including the digestive, circulatory and immune systems, are compromised when the lymphatic system is bogged down with excess toxins and unable to function as a result of insufficient body movement. It's easy to see that all of the systems are interrelated.

We all want to have beautiful skin, and in order for our skin to have that special glow that we all associate with a healthy body, it is important to detoxify the lymphatic system. Seventy percent of the capillaries that carry this "dirty" lymph from each cell and outward to the lymph nodes are located near the surface of the skin.[6] By keeping toxins to a minimum through a healthy diet, and combining this lifestyle with a daily regimen of body movement through exercise, dry skin brushing, and massage, the lymphatic system will benefit. Lastly, another important part of any healthy regimen for lymphatic cleansing would include drinking at least three liters of water per day.

---

[6] Lymph Notes. http://www.lymphnotes.com/article.php/id/151/

How Do I Skin Brush?

Just as the Japanese performed their loofa scrubbing before entering the hot spring baths, today we perform for ten minutes *prior* to a bath or shower, once or even twice per day. The routine is simple enough for anyone. Using gentle, sweeping strokes, it is recommended to brush as follows:

1. Up both legs, from ankles to knees, and from knees to hips (90 seconds each leg, total approximately 3 minutes).

2. Up both arms, from wrists elbows, and from elbows to shoulders (90 seconds each arm, total approximately 3 minutes).

3. Down the neck, up the abdomen and back towards the thoracic cavity. (Approximately 2 minutes each per front and back).

NOTE: If you have irritated, red, bruised, burned, or otherwise sensitive skin, these areas must be avoided when skin brushing. Also, it is never recommended to perform skin brushing on the areas of the face. Long, gentle strokes are typically used, while once participants are more used to the sensation, they often tend to use a little bit more pressure. Some people like to target certain "problem" areas using a slightly more pressured, circular stroke; brushing for another minute or so, on the areas of the buttocks, stomach, and thighs. To finish, use sweeping, straight strokes towards the abdomen, (because this is where all of the waste product makes its exit out from the body). Be gentle and careful to avoid over-exfoliation, which causes the skin to be red, irritated, and open to pathogens and debris.

It is also recommended that whenever possible, an epsom salt bath is used after skin brushing in order to further cleanse and nourish the body through the circulation of lymph. (Another newer technique called salt-glow therapy is being increasingly used for additional stimulation of the lymphatic system following skin brushing treatments by massage therapists and naturopaths for treating their patients.

Information about salt-glow therapy can readily be accessed on the web, for example, at massagetherapy.com.)

Many people also finish their lymphatic cleansing routine in the bath or shower with a cold rinse, to continue to circulate the lymph throughout the body.[7] It is believed that the morning is the best time to skin brush because toxins are released while we are sleeping, and need to be flushed out. Throughout the day, other activities that stimulate lymphatic cleansing are: (1) deep diaphragmatic breathing,[8] (2) at least 5 minutes a day of jumping on a mini-trampoline or jumping rope, or other exercise, and (3) therapeutic massage.

---

[7] Center for Lymphatic Health. http://www.lymphatichealth.com/skin-brushing/
[8] Natural News. http://www.naturalnews.com/041284_lymphological_birthing_childbirth_deep_breathing.html

Why Should I Skin Brush Daily?

The capillaries of the lymphatic system that are found primarily just beneath the surface of the skin, together with the kidneys, lungs, large intestines and liver, are a part of the excretory system. This is of course a system that removes excess, unnecessary materials from the body, in the forms of gas, liquid, and solid wastes, "so as to maintain homeostasis… and prevent damage to the body."[9]

Skin brushing daily feels invigorating and clarifying. It's a good time to do some stretches, clear out the gunk in your junk (so to speak) and get ready for the day. But more specifically, skin brushing has numerous documented benefits, and these are the 7 reasons why dry skin brushing daily is a valuable part of a healthy routine.

---

[9] Wikipedia.
http://en.wikipedia.org/wiki/Excretory_system#Defecation

1. **The lymphatic system carries nutrients to every cell in the body**

   The lymph fluid breaks down digestible fats and fat-soluble vitamins from the digestive system in the lower intestines and carries these nutrients from the lower extremities, through the pelvis and thoracic cavity, to the arms and finally the heart.

2. **The lymphatic system carries away toxins from every cell in the body, leaving our bodies in a more energized and youthful state.**

Toxins from the outside world, such as microorganisms and other living particles,[10] as well as byproducts of joint and muscle use, (such as arthritic and lactic acids, and even cancer cells),[11] are carried out of our cells through the lymphatic system[12], minimizing damage to the body, and are filtered through a network of over 500 lymph nodes. Seventy percent of the capillaries that carry this "dirty" lymph from each cell and outward to the lymph nodes are located near the surface of the skin.[13] An example many people think of is the visible swollen lymph nodes we often see on either side of someone's neck, just below their ear, when they aren't feeling well.

---

[10] National Cancer Institute.
http://training.seer.cancer.gov/anatomy/lymphatic/
[11] Wikipedia. http://en.wikipedia.org/wiki/Lymph
[12] National Institute of Health.
http://www.ncbi.nlm.nih.gov/pmc/articles/PMC2755111/
[13] Lymph Notes. http://www.lymphnotes.com/article.php/id/151/

In cases where the lymphatic system is not in peak operating condition, the muscles will have a tendency to tighten up due to the build-up of lactic acid and excess fluid around the cells.[14] By stimulating this system and removing unnecessary fluid buildup, and ridding the body of foreign matter and invaders such as bacteria and cancer cells[15], the body is left with more energy to use on other areas, such as cell rejuvenation, nervous system activities, and digestion.

---

[14] Natural News.
http://www.naturalnews.com/041284_lymphological_birthing_childbirth_deep_breathing.html#ixzz2t18QzEli
[15] National Institute of Health.
http://www.nlm.nih.gov/medlineplus/ency/article/002247.htm

3. **The lymphatic system creates antibodies, which are the cells that fight infections and keep us healthy.**

The lymphatic system is part of the immune system. The organs of the immune system include: tonsils and adenoids, lymph nodes, lymphatic vessels, thymus, spleen, appendix, and bone marrow.

The cells that are created in the thymus and bone marrow are able to determine whether a virus, bacteria, parasite, cancer cell, or another person's tissue has entered the bloodstream. These foreign invaders are then carried through the lymphatic fluid to the lymph nodes, where they are filtered out and targeted for attack by antibodies.[16]

---

[16] U.S. Government. http://aids.gov/hiv-aids-basics/just-diagnosed-with-hiv-aids/hiv-in-your-body/immune-system-101/

4. The lymphatic system does not have a pumping mechanism of its own.

Lymph is initially part of blood, but as it flows through the body, lymph slowly separates, taking hazardous substances with it and filtering these substances through the lymph nodes. Unlike blood, lymph does not have a central pump, relying instead on a series of other bodily functions to circulate the lymph through the thoracic cavity and back to the heart, where it is recirculated.[17] Lymph can be found all over the body, in fact, if you have ever had a cut that oozed out clear fluid, this was lymph.

---

[17] All Health Studio. http://allhealthstudio.com/the-lymphatic-system.php

5. Skin brushing eases a number of other ailments.

People attribute a range of ailments to a failing or sluggish lymphatic system. A blocked lymphatic system can be a cause of allergies, frequent colds, chronic sinusitis, high blood pressure, lack of energy, weight gain, joint pain, and headaches. People who have had their lymph nodes removed as a form of cancer treatment often suffer from lymphedema, which is the swelling of the affected arm or area. Lymphedema is caused by a blockage in the lymphatic system, which prevents the lymphatic fluid from draining properly.[18]

Skin brushing at least five times per week, preferably in the morning, (as toxins have a tendency to accumulate as we sleep), helps to eliminate these symptoms. Of importance is that it is often thought

---

[18] Mayo Clinic. http://www.mayoclinic.org/diseases-conditions/lymphedema/basics/definition/CON-20025603

that about a month of routine skin brushing is needed before noticeable results are experienced.[19]

---

[19] Gargulinski, R. http://www.livestrong.com/article/319521-does-brushing-cellulite-really-help/ August 16, 2013.

6. Skin brushing helps tighten skin through improving circulation.

Whether as result of rapid weight loss, or as a regular sign of aging, our skin occasionally needs help with retaining its firmness. Ask anyone who has ever seen cellulite in the mirror- this is one of the scarier issues of aging, because so many times even the most physically active people have an element of cellulite on their body. Cellulite is fat underneath the skin that presses against connective tissue, causing the dimpling effect.[20] Cellulite most often affects women, with 80% of women noticing cellulite on their body at some point. Toxins are stored in the fat cells of the body, which can show up as cellulite. While genetics, hormones, and other factors also contribute to the amount of cellulite on a person's body, a sluggish lymphatic system is often involved with this unsightly condition. Skin brushing provides an excellent mechanism for the body to remove the waste products that are associated with cellulite, by carrying

---

[20] http://www.webmd.com/beauty/cellulite/cellulite-causes-and-treatments February 9, 2014

these toxins to the primary areas of elimination: the kidneys, lungs, colon and skin.[21]

---

[21] Gargulinski, R. http://www.livestrong.com/article/319521-does-brushing-cellulite-really-help/ August 16, 2013.

7. Skin brushing can help you lose weight.

By aiding in the removal of waste from the body through improving the lymphatic drainage, and the resulting effects on the digestive and elimination systems, skin brushing helps people lose weight.[22] While this is not a comprehensive weight loss system in and of itself, it is an aide in the efforts of stimulating the elimination system.

---

[22] Livestrong. http://www.livestrong.com/article/297902-lymphatic-massage-for-weight-loss/

What Other Elements of a Skin Care Routine Are Key?

Many people believe the chemicals in conventional skin care products are dangerous to our bodies because of the rate of absorption through the skin. By some estimates, chemicals in our skin may be absorbed into our bodies even faster than water. Using natural skin care products that contain as few ingredients as possible helps minimize the contact we have with large molecules of various chemical compounds that are added to our cosmetics today. Hundreds of chemicals have been researched in their effects on the human body, including: butyl paraben, sodium laurel sulfate, sodium laureth sulfate, fragrances, mineral oil, polyethylene glycol (PEG), butylene glycol, DEA (diethanolamine), MEA (monoethanolamine), TEA (triethanolamine), triclosan, and FD&C Color Pigments. The simple answer is that reaction rates, if any, to these compounds will vary from person to person, and as with any process that occurs over time, it is very difficult to clearly pinpoint how much of an effect our individual, daily routines have… But it is still better to be safe than sorry!

Note: This information is for educational purposes only and is not intended as a prescription. Each person is advised to consult their health care provider whenever trying a new routine. Never skin brush irritated, red, scabbed, or broken skin. Also, do not brush directly in the eyes, ears, nose, or mouth.

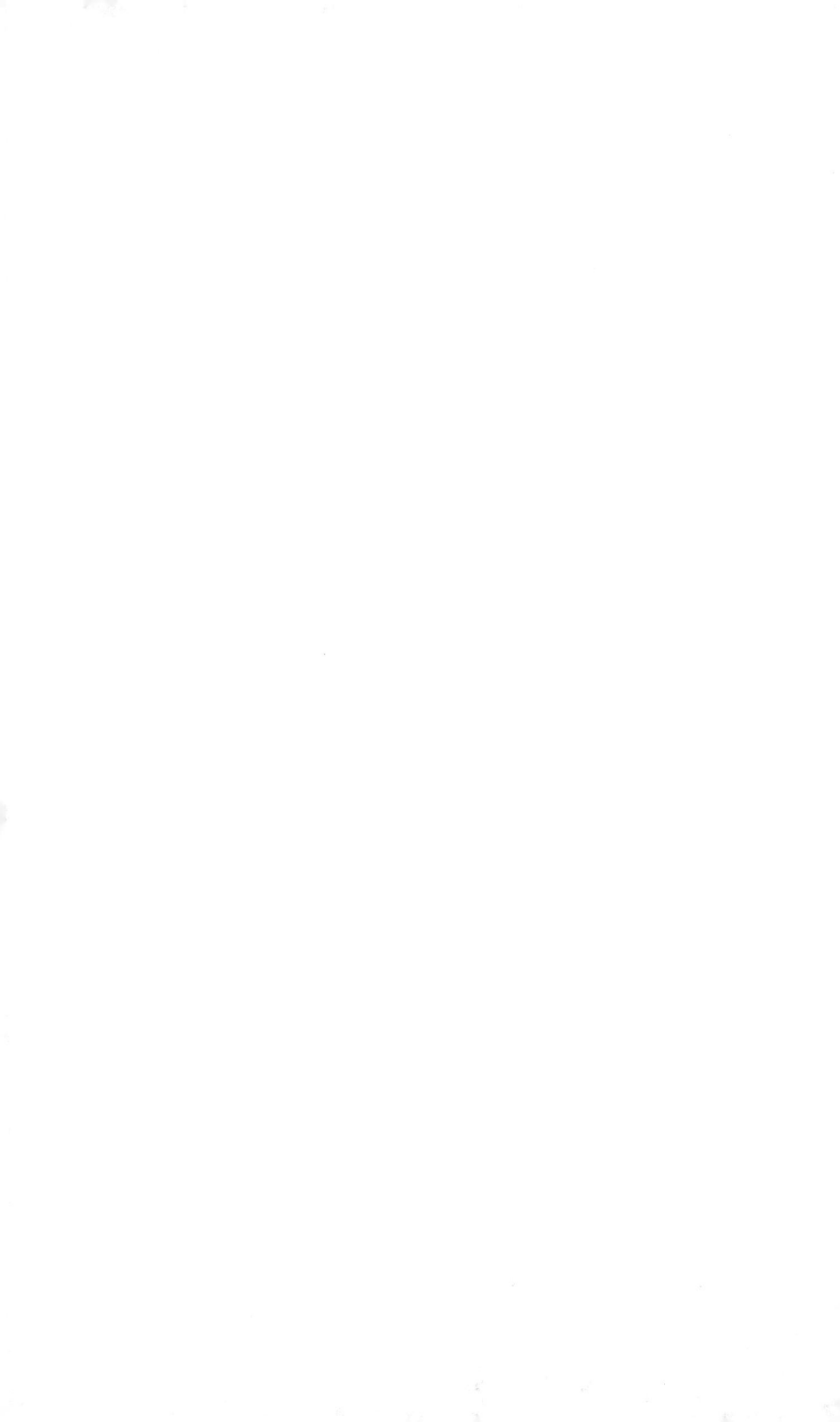